Walk By Faith: God's Divine Interception

By: Taneya Pair

Walk By Faith: God's Divine Interception

By: Taneya Pair

Copyright © 2022 by Taneya Pair

Printed in the United States of America.

ISBN-13: 978-0-578-29304-2

Book Cover: Jennee Lamb, Master Developer of Greater Good Development Group
www.GGDevelopmentGroup.com
Jennee@GreaterGoodDevelopmentGroup.com

Photographer: Shawn Turrentine
Art Trends, LLC
ArtTrendsPhoto@gmail.com www.arttrendsllc.com

Book Editor: Shanice L. Stewart of Red Ink Editing Services RedInkEditing2017@gmail.com

Contact Information:

Website: www.TaneyaMonese.com
Email: Contact@TaneyaMonese.com
Instagram: TaneyaMonese
Facebook: Taneya Pair

Dedication

This book is dedicated to my late Mentor Dr. Reverend Yasmine Bell, Friend Dr. Nicole King and Mrs. Laverne Talley. I kept my promise and by the grace of God this the book is finished.

From Labor to Reward.

Thank you for your encouragement, correction, and patience.

Love, Tee

Acknowledgements

Thank you to my Lord and Savior Jesus Christ and the direction of the Holy Spirit for the inspiration and guidance to complete this book. Many may not understand the power and significance of the Holy Spirit. However, there are decisions and insights that the human mind can't understand alone. The decision to have a mammogram referral written for a 32-year-old patient, without any history of breast cancer can only be directed by the Holy Spirit Himself. I respect all other beliefs and religions. However, this is my testimony and understanding of how my journey began.

To my late amazing mentor Reverend Dr. Yasmine Bell. Thank you for the assurance and encouragement you gave me throughout my life's journey. You lived a life of service which was full of excellence, humility, and commitment to the purpose God placed you on this earth to fulfill. Your love and wisdom will continue to inspire me. Thank you for being supportive when I first discussed writing this book months before you passed away. You were the light and fire that kept me going. I will do what you've always told me which was, "Go out and do great things." I will keep my promise.

To the church that prepared and watched me grow into a woman of faith, First Baptist Church of Highland Park. Thank you for the continuous prayer, love, and support given throughout my journey. I am forever grateful for the heart of family and servanthood that the ministry pours into others. Dr. Henry P. Davis III, Dr. Weptanomah Davis and the entire FBHP family, thank you for everything.

To Ray, my first mentor. Life has not dealt me the greatest card in life. However, in every moment you were there to step in and help me strategically play every card I was dealt through the wisdom of God. Thank you for building my foundation and piecing together a broken girl, who just wanted to love Jesus. You are a profound woman of God, whose legacy is living and is currently moving within my life and others. Thank you for your sacrifice and grace. The years of impartations from you have begun to come to fruition and God is just getting started. You will benefit from the fruits of your labor.

To my mentor, Pastor Victoria Harris, your push is special and unique. A trailblazer will always push you to your greatest potential and will not stop until you build up traction and momentum. Thank you for being the fire, strength, and influence that I needed. Life can feel unfair at times, but I thank you for lifting my head in the worst and greatest of times. The day I had my biopsy, you did not hesitate to jump in to support me and that love has not changed. Thank you for being Lady Fire and imparting grace and strength within me. Thank you for praying with me and walking with me as you have. You are and will always be a blessing to my life. Thank you!

To Ms. Peggy Kirk (Ma Peggy), through it all in the highs and lows you have remained by my side. Thank you for your teaching and talks of prayer, obedience to the Father and womanhood. You have been one of the greatest gifts to my life. Thank you for imparting the wisdom of God and His word into my life. In every decision I made throughout this journey, you supported me along with the way and I thank you.

To Kingdom Deliverance Ministry International, Apostle Jimmie C Thompson, Prophet Natalie Thompson and family, thank you so much for your encouragement, support, and wisdom. I love you all greatly.

To Nurse Practitioner Jaki Bradley, thank you for saving my life and in essence, being used by God as the watchman who prevented the cancer from being a late catch. God used you by the direction of the Holy Spirit to save my life and for that, I thank you so much.

To Dr. McSwain and Dr. Lenert, the phenomenal duo Wonder Women Team of George Washington University Hospital, thank you for saving my life and creating a calm and joyful journey throughout this time. Thank you for your patience, care, and love. You two are a dynamic duo and I thank God for placing you two in my life. Thank you.

To my great friend, prayer warrior, advisor, sister, editor, and the one who has walked with me since the year I rededicated my life to Christ, Mrs. Shanice L. Stewart. You are a beacon of light, joy, and hope in my life. Thank you for being the one to remind me that I had a purpose and voice. Thank you for creating the space with *Share Your Testimony* which allowed me to share my story with others when I believed I had nothing to share. Life has not been the same since that day and I am thankful for you and your friendship.

To my siblings, thank you. To Kayla (MyKayKay), receiving the news probably was not easy for you but I thank you for remaining strong for everyone. For you to be the first person I saw the moment I opened my eyes after my first surgery, along with a cactus plant and Victoria Secret's gift card for my new bras blessed me. I love you all so much.

To my family, grandmothers, grandfathers, dad, mom, uncles, aunts, and cousins thank you for the roles that you served whether it near or far within this journey. The love and support was felt and it helped me more than you know.

To my village and host of friends, your prayers, support, encouragement, and accountability allowed this project to come to fruition. The many times that I wanted to give up, you all kept me going. The many times I allowed the matters of life to consume me, you pulled me up. I am eternally grateful for you all. As my brothers and sisters, thank you all so much.

To my mentees, there is nothing that life will bring that you can't face. With God, all things are possible. Strength is built through movement and no matter what life brings, don't stop moving. You are amazing and blessed to succeed in graced in life. I will walk with you each step of the way and be your biggest cheerleader and accountability, partner. I love you. Thank you for encouraging me to be a better me for you. Thank you for trusting God in me with you.

Foreword

In my 27 years as a Nurse Practitioner, I have had to share unpleasant news with patients. However, once I accepted God in my life & I became a bold Christian. It is to Him that I give honor and glory for the privilege of caring for His people.

You see, God could have placed Taneya in the exam room with any provider, but He chose me to be His instrument that faithful day. What was interesting was that I felt as if I was comforting an old friend. In fact, we both felt comfortable that day sharing our faith, praying, crying, and asking God to give us the strength to get through that hard conversation. God had prepared both of us for this day. We know that God allows us to experience trials that refine our faith. Holding onto that faith was not going to be easy for Taneya, as she maneuvered the medical system.

When Taneya found herself in the midst of this trial, she could have been fixated on the diagnosis and lost perspective. Instead, she chose the alternative and remembered what James said, "Consider it pure joy, my brothers and sisters, whenever you face trials of many kinds, because you know that the testing of your faith produces perseverance." James 1: 2-3 NIV And boy did she preserver!

We had faith that she would get through this trial, because we serve a faithful God. We knew that by faith the woman with the issue of blood was healed; by faith Job endured illness and losses and was healed (Mathew 15:23); by faith a blind man received his sight (Mark 10:52); by faith Jesus healed ten lepers (Luke 17-11-19) and by faith Taneya endured the cancer diagnosis, treatment, and healing.

Some would ask, why did God allow this to happen? The answer is simple... to share the good news with you! God will use anyone and any situation for His purpose. My prayer is that this book will encourage you to draw closer to God, as you *Walk by Faith* through your valley and experience God's faithfulness and joy.

PS: Taneya, you have said on more than one occasion that I saved your life...No, God saved your life so the world would see His glory.

I leave you with this prayer: *Lord, thank you for the refining our faith through trials. Thank you for using Taneya to touch the saved and unsaved. Strengthen their faith so they can endure. You are a good Father. Thank you for your grace, mercy, kindness and yes...our trials, in the mighty name of Jesus! Amen.*

Jaki Bradley, MSS, MSN, CRNP

Table of Contents

Divine Interception

I dedicate this time of sharing my story with you. Whether you are a warrior, who has entered your journey of breast cancer, a family member or significant other, a co-worker, or a friend who desires to read firsthand of what a person goes through, this is for you. My prayer is that this book allows you to be present and an effective support system to someone experiencing this journey. As a millennial single woman with no children and never married, the last thing that I would want to hear was unexpected news regarding my health. I am not sure if you are in your 20s, 30s, 40s, 50s, 60s, 70s, 80s, or 90s, but can you imagine pondering about how you would hope or expect your life to be, and without notice, you are hit with something that could change your life greatly? You find yourself faced with having to make serious life decisions that will determine the outcome of your life (honestly life/death), meanwhile, you desire to focus on other things that you enjoy doing. You now have to prepare for a moment in your life, where you can't invest your time into living without a care in the world. You are now forced to shift your focus, because your health and future is dependent on your decisions.

As a 32-year-old woman, the only thing I thought about during that time was the success of my career. In a person's 30s, most people are focused on whether or not to continue education, build wealth and finances, travel and explore the world, build and/or raise a family, build relationships or meet new people, and discover life as an adult. Most times you think about your next steps in life. Without expectancy comes a moment where you receive news that you were not hoping for. There are going to come times in your life when you receive news that can either make or break your faith. Throughout this journey, I've learned a mind is a powerful tool. Your mind will guide you through areas that seem impossible, challenging, and also intimidating. Here's a blessing; when your heart and mind align together, your faith can be cultivated and developed.

Here's my story and I hope my words will bring encouragement to you as you go through or enter your journey.

22

Mammogram at 32? Why? What caused me to get a mammogram?

In May 2020, I changed my insurance and decided to meet with a new primary care physician and a therapist. I've always had great health and would go as needed outside of my regular yearly exams. However, I went through several moments of depression that I decided that it was time for me to meet with a therapist under this new insurance. So, I decided to contact my primary care to schedule an appointment along with an appointment with a new therapist. Let me pause for a second, God will allow moments to enter into your life without you even knowing why to prepare you from a life-changing situation that will soon arise. I push the importance of having a relationship with God. God knows your thoughts and body more than you do. So, why not build a relationship with

Him? I tell you the truth, I probably would be in Lord knows what kind of condition physically, mentally, emotionally, and spiritually right now had I not made my initial appointments with my therapist and primary care doctor.

I knew there was a change that needed to happen in my life, and I was determined to figure it out. In May and June, I experienced three deaths, and this was during the time of COVID-19. In the month of May, I honestly asked God, where was He? I noticed that I continued to go into moments of depression, and the consistency was like none other. Hence why I decided to reach out to find a new therapist. I had no idea that my life was preparing to take a turn that I was not prepared for.

So, why did I get the mammogram? Mid May after finding the number for my new doctor and before making an appointment, I decided to do a self-breast exam. Prior to this day, I did not perform regular self-breast exams and would only do them once randomly every other year. Breast Health was important to me as it should've been. During this self-breast exam, I felt a lump on my left breast. The lump wasn't alarming to me because I was told by my previous physician, whom I've had for years that I had fibrocystic breast. In October 2019, I had an ultrasound done because I was concerned, and the results showed that the cyst in my breast was benign. After discovering the lump in May 2020, I thought to myself, "Ok, this is a new doctor let me be sure to bring this up during our first appointment." If you are anything like me, I am bringing every problem I can think of that's wrong with me during my appointment.

Here I am with this new doctor, and she tells me about herself, and we discovered that we were familiar with each other's church, and we began to build a rapport. My doctor examined my breast and asked me about my cancer history within my family. I informed her that I was told two weeks before my appointment, that a family member of mine was examined for ovarian cancer, and I had yet to receive the reports from that exam. It was at that moment that I believe God's Divine Interception was coming into play on the field of my journey. I am not a sports fanatic at all. I love watching the game of football, but I don't understand it. However, follow me as I walk through this divine interception play. It is moments like this that while we are remaining obedient to following the pull, move, or instructions of God is when He is already strategically placing angels and in place to intercept and block every arrow, dart, tackle, and blow that will derail you from living the life that God has for you. The purpose of any negative thing that comes into your life is to knock you off course, so as long as the ball is in the attacker's hand, he's running down the field in hopes of scoring a goal or touch down...

follow me for a second, because I'm going somewhere. What I believe is, God will allow the enemy to have the ball in his hand. He's running and moving *like* the Most Valuable Player. Keyword *Like* but in reality, he's not. This reminds me of 1 Peter 5:8, "Stay alert! Watch out for your great enemy, the devil. He prowls around LIKE a roaring lion, looking for someone to devour." **So, here comes the opposing team Like the most valuable players running with my future, destiny, purpose, choices, calling, power, and all in his hand ready to score a touchdown, and here comes God with His mighty hand**. God places His angels on the field in place for the interception. That's for you! God will allow the enemy to move like he has power, but he doesn't. What I want you to know is just because things seem contrary to what you believe your life to be, that does not solidify the final point and story of your life. God will be exalted over everything that comes into your life. Your challenges have a purpose. Your setbacks have a purpose, and the times when you have to ask God where He is has a purpose. You must be built up in your faith, in your purpose, and in the understanding of who you are in Him. Much of the time discovering this happens during contrary moments. What do the football people say, "INO" short for interception…. I think at least.

After sharing the information with my new primary care, she completed an exam that appeared to be normal to me. Minutes later, she typed a referral and stated, "I want you to get a mammogram of both breasts." I was shocked and confused at that moment. I thought to myself, "Huh? Women don't get breast mammograms until age 40." The referral was odd to me. However, I scheduled the appointment for June 5, 2020. After I completed my mammogram exam, I noticed that I was waiting in my doctor's office longer than I expected. I was certain that this appointment was going to be 45 minutes to an hour at the most. Instead, I was there for two hours. The technician completed the mammogram and an ultrasound, then recommended that I receive further testing. I was informed that the techs noticed calcification pieces in my right breast. May I remind you that I originally went to the doctor with concerns about my left breast. After the mammogram, the images showed the left breast was fine. The right breast on the other hand, which was not aching, painless, and lump free was the breast where the calcification was discovered. At this point, I am nervous and shocked, because I was expecting to have this quick exam, go home and enjoy the remainder of my day. After receiving my referral for my breast biopsy, I immediately texted my mentor Pastor Victoria Venable and told her what happened. The text followed with encouraging words and her stating that she would be there with me no matter what.

As I gathered my belongings, I headed to the receptionist desk. The receptionist who provided me with my papers and directions to the office for my biopsy in the sweetest voice said, "Everything will be ok, but make sure to schedule your appointment." There was this unexplainable peace this older woman had with her that comforted me for that moment. When I sat in my car, I cried because I never had to go through tests or had any health concerns throughout my entire life. This was the beginning of a new life for me, and I had no idea of what would transpire after this.

Timely Instant Decisions

I decided to call the facility and schedule the biopsy appointment. I was nervous and honestly intimidated once I arrived. My biopsy was completed on June 25, 2020.

May I be candid with you? My biopsy appointment was during the height of the Black Lives Matter movement, racial injustices, and inequality throughout the nation. Personally, my anxiety and frustration were at a level that I'd never imagined with Caucasians.... Hey, don't close my book after that statement because that was my truth. *However, in all of my anxieties, fears, concerns, and lack of trust with Caucasians, let alone in the medical field and trusting them with my life, this journey allowed me to let God heal me of that very fear.* Guess what? Each medical staff that walked with me through this journey were all Caucasian. That was not due to my personal choice, but God's plan of Divine Interception. The fears that I had with receiving medical assistance from Caucasians began many years ago, as far back as high school. For many years, I would intentionally pick doctors that looked like me, and not because of their credentials, background, or status. I made the decisions because of my biases and fears of the medical world and physicians who did not look like me. I would even side-eye the Caucasian front desk representative wondering if they were trying to mix up my files or do anything other than their job of effectively assisting me. My fears and lack of trust were that bad.

So, had I not focused on what mattered the most, which was my health and walking and believing by faith that God had everything under control, I probably would have been the cause of my cancer becoming worse than it was. My ignorance would have kept me in bondage and sick, because of my thoughts. Throughout this journey, I had to mature more than I was as it pertained to my medical decision making. **I had to deal with a lot of internal issues when it came to trust and medicine to save my life.**

So, here I am sitting in the waiting room, at my biopsy appointment with breast cancer awareness pictures, and a wall decal that read, "Believe, Courage, Faith, Hope, Peace, Strength, Cure, Love" with a pink breast cancer ribbon in the middle. While meeting with the surgeon, I was informed that there was a tracker that would go into my breast, and at that moment, I almost canceled the entire appointment. I said, "A tracker?" and as I asked questions, the responses were so vague that my lack of trust increased even more. I respectfully said that I would like to return to my doctor's office and discuss everything with her. I felt uncomfortable and the main reason once again was my lack of trust in Caucasian doctors. The process of overcoming that fear and the maturity God began in me, started during that very moment. I asked questions and I felt as if the doctor was not patient with me or cared for helping me process the information he provided. I then decided to leave. As I left out of the building and returned to my car with my dad who drove with me to the appointment. I shared my concerns with my dad, and he supported my decision. My dad and I sat in the car for about five minutes which felt like 15 minutes, as I felt the urgency to go back into the office to have the biopsy completed. I informed my dad that I was just going to return to the facility, complete the biopsy and get it over with. I returned to the facility and proceeded with the biopsy. The procedure was uncomfortable; however, I knew that I had to do what I had to do to see what was going on. I was numbed in my right breast, which was painful. The numbing medicine wasn't strong enough, and I felt each pull of my tissue from the six samples that were removed. The nurse who held my hand asked the doctor to numb me again and I told them not to because the needle was just as painful. As I went through with the mini procedure, the nurse held my hand and sang a hymnal that I was familiar with (I can't remember what it was to this day). She was another angel of peace on earth. *After the six tissue samples were removed, the physician checked the monitor and the nurse said, "If this comes back as what we think it (cancer) is, this is the earliest catch we've ever seen."* At that moment walking by faith began to develop, and it developed in a space that I never visited before. One thing about faith and when facing an unfamiliar moment in your life, your level and depth of faith will guide you and keep you. You must decide if you're going to believe the facts and outcome of whatever the outcome could be. Or are you going to walk by faith and not by what you see, and know that no matter what you are going to fight this? After the biopsy appointment, I waited two weeks until I received my results which were the longest two weeks I've ever experienced.

The Call

I received a call from my primary care on the morning of July 6, 2020, and she asked me if I was home alone. The moment she asked the question, I knew something was wrong. I informed her that I was at my mother's house, as I prepared myself mentally to receive whatever she had to tell me. Within seconds she broke the news to me. And as I am writing to you, my reader, I am getting emotional just thinking about it. She stated that the results came back as cancerous, and it was in its early stage. I immediately went numb, and I began to hyperventilate. My body was there, but my mind and awareness of where I was and what was going on at that time, were frozen. Though it felt like everything sat at a standstill, I recall my physician asking to speak with my mom. I gave my mother the phone and I completely phased out. Meaning I was frozen and could not articulate or understand anything that my mom was saying, as she spoke with my doctor on the phone. I just sat on the edge of my mom's bed, turned my head, and stared out the window, which filled my mother's room with light from the bright sun. My mom ended the call and **I asked with tears in my eyes, "Why me?"** Her response was something that I wasn't expecting because my mother isn't one of many words. My mom said, **"God picks and chooses who He wants to use for a reason and He chose you because you have a voice."** This statement stuck with me, but I had no idea that those words would help me get through the next months of my life. The next few months stretched my faith and confidence in what God was doing within me.

Week 1: After the Call

My first week was not easy at all. I cried I prayed, I screamed, I was fearful, and I was very transparent with God throughout this time. However, during this first week, I reminded myself that I had two options in this situation: I had to Fight or Flight. Fighting meant I had to build up my trust in God through prayer, educate myself on the condition, conduct my research, and put things in a place mentally, physically, and spiritually. I wanted to put my faith into action by holding up my end of this journey. Fighting also meant I had to walk by faith. Flight meant that I could've allowed depression, worry, and anxiety to get the best of me. I did not want to settle in defeat without trying to fight. This is coming from someone who was spiraling in depression one month before this moment (which felt like a blow to the gut) asking God where He was after losing three people who were close to them during the pandemic. However, I believe that God was with me in this because had He left me, the pressure would have destroyed me. I would not be able to write to you and I probably would not have the health that I have today if I allowed depression to consume me when I received the news of my cancer diagnosis. I decided to fight!

In this journey, you will learn to fight along with discovering the importance of knowing that you are the patient and are a priority along with finding your voice to advocate for yourself.

The first surgeon I met at a local hospital was not patient with me, my questions were rushed, and she said something that caused me to look at her sideways and made me question her professionalism. She did not give me time to process all of the information that she gave me regarding the diagnosis, and she was trying to rush the surgery immediately. There were discussions about my surgery date and she and her assistant continued to call me regarding the date, and the calls made me feel uncomfortable. I did not feel supported, and her engagements and conversations with me seemed like a business meeting. The conversations felt as if it was a lack of her understanding that this is a very delicate and serious matter. At the time, I was a young patient who had never experienced hospitalization or surgeries, let alone cancer. My wisdom for you is whatever you do, ask questions during your visits, and do not leave until some of the answers have been explained to you.

When people first think about cancer, they think their life is over, and everything regarding their life is doomed. At times people who aren't personally dealing with cancer, at times will assume the worst more than the person who has it. I want you, my reader to understand that this is a serious and delicate journey. And anyone who does not respect that, does not need to have direct access to you within the journey. Anyone meaning, friends, family, and also medical staff. So, in my encounters with this surgeon, instead of settling with feeling like I'm just a regular patient or a regular diagnosis, I had to stand up for myself. I decided to seek a different surgeon at a local well-known hospital, who turned out to be the most phenomenal surgeon. I also believe I had and have the most phenomenal team in the world at George Washington Hospital. I am so grateful for the staff, team, and nurses because they walked with me each step of the way. In life, we must make decisions that reflect where we want to go in life. I believe that I had to step out of my comfort zone to receive true strength, unity, and clarity in the time that I was facing. You have to be secure in your decisions and take time to process why you are making the decisions and where it stems from. Looking back on my decisions and biases with the medical field, there's no telling what dysfunction and destruction my fears would have caused me. This decision was just for me, because my plans and ways of doing things regarding my choices of who I wanted to be cared by, wasn't God's plans. This decision was the best that I could've made during this time of my journey.

Find Your Voice

One thing that I want to share with you is: you have to find your voice. When I say your voice I mean your specific voice, not the voice of your family members, your friends, your significant other; you have to find your voice. Why? Your voice will carry you throughout this journey, your voice will give you the confidence to say, "I don't like this" and "I'm uncomfortable with how I'm being serviced or cared for" especially when it comes to your appointments. **You have to learn to speak up!** You have to discover your voice in your voice. And why do I say that? I say this because you will have people who love you, who may genuinely have your best interest at heart. However, you cannot move at the tone and the rhythm of their drum. A lot of people may think they know what's best for you, but it could be stressful for you during this time.

When I received my diagnosis, I did not tell everybody. I did not tell all of my friends or associates, I didn't tell all of my family members, and I didn't tell even my closest friends. Why? The reason why I didn't tell everyone, is because everybody does not need to be a part of those most fragile moments of your journey when you are trying to process everything.

Some people have faith in God until a serious situation arises that may test their faith. If their faith isn't strong enough to hold them up plus you, it may crumble your foundation. Their faith may waiver or may even be at a standstill and lifeless. You don't need anyone who exhibits those behaviors around you. You have to be careful who you talk about this journey with early on. Depression is real when receiving a diagnosis of cancer, because most people instantly assume death. Those same thoughts will find their way to consume you with fear and place you in a space of isolation. If you were already fighting off all these thoughts of fear and depression, the last thing that you need is not strong enough people to speak power into your situation and your life. Be mindful of who's around you as you discover your voice. Know that your thoughts and feelings matter. Your voice of strength will build you up as you go throughout your journey, and it will also be a voice for someone else who is going through the journey that you have already overcome. I know because I'm here with you.

You have to be mindful of who's asking too many questions. Sometimes too many questions can be overwhelming, especially when you are processing matters that you are unfamiliar with. You will have moments when you need to take a step back and breathe alone. Moments of inhaling and exhaling releases were frequent for me. Give yourself the right and luxuries of having time to yourself to just breathe. People can create a space of anxiety and depression that's not even at the level that the person facing cancer is experiencing. People will transfer their worries and fears of cancer to you when your levels weren't high as their level of fear. **Sometimes you have to tell people, "Give me some time to process through this".** You don't need people around you who live in fear and doubt. You don't need negative people around you who are going to speak what they think is best for you, especially if they are inconsistent with their own mental, emotional, physical, and spiritual health. When I first received my diagnosis, there were only four people who knew and they were strong men and women in faith. There's nothing against anyone who I didn't tell during the first few months of my journey. However, I had to be strategic and careful with whom I told. I trusted the wisdom of God within these individuals and knew that they were not going to allow me to settle, fail, run or hide from this illness. First and foremost, you

54

must develop a relationship with God and trust the wisdom He gives you during this process. You have to align your faith to the fact that God said that He would never leave you alone and that He is omnipresent. Your faith in God's plan has to be in alignment with every person throughout this journey, including your medical team. Pay attention to your medical team. You will know you have a good team when they are patient and consistent in their communication with you. The team is reachable. The nurses and assistants are attentive to you. Pay attention to how the staff conducts themselves and assists you during your appointment visits. Pay attention to how your doctor talks to you, their tone and how they focus their attention to you. You are a priority and as their patient during your appointment, you are top priority. So, find your voice. Your voice speaks volumes. Your voice is priority. Your voice is needed.

Priority Over Pleasure

During this time, you'll discover how certain things in your life can weigh you down along with discovering balance. Your happiness, joy, peace, healing, and your life are all priorities. When it came to this journey, I had understood that I was entering into a space of learning how to put myself first. In learning how to put me first, I discovered what brought me happiness. There's a difference between joy and happiness. Joy is something eternal that is within you, and it can't be taken from you no matter what comes and goes within your life. However, happiness is temporary. Happiness is found in things and even moments that are temporary and serve their perfect purpose for that moment. The cycle of discovered happiness will continue to appear at different moments in your life and within different tangible things. For me, I had to get rid of the extra unnecessary emotional, mental, and spiritual weight that I was carrying. I had to get rid of what may sound simple to some, but it was something that was a part of my stress that I had to get rid of; an almost 5-year car note that was never going anywhere. I stepped out on faith and God blessed me to get rid of that car and purchase my dream car. I thank God that I had the finances to put a down payment on my brand new 2020 Ford Mustang, two weeks before my 33rd birthday. However, I didn't just stop there. **The tangible happiness was nice. However, I had to deal with the spiritual baggage that I carried around.** I had to discover the offenses and stresses that I held onto for years with people. I had to release them for me to be released of the weight that I carried for years. I had to release my hurt in order for me to walk in freedom. So, my focus was to contact those who I had offenses with because one thing that you don't want to do is go into this new journey and still hold onto stresses that have absolutely no significance within your life at this moment. You are a warrior, who has decided to live. You have made a significant decision to put yourself first. So, that goes with everything else that's outside of you. **If it is not aligned with what brings you happiness, or of excitement and motivation that empowers you to what keeps you going through this journey with clarity, it must go!** That includes people, places, and things. The offenses that I held onto, developed due to disappointments I held onto for years. The hurt that I held onto was with family, and current and past friends. I held onto offenses because I dealt with a lot of rejection, disappointment, and feeling ostracized. Many of my challenges stemmed from battles in my childhood and teenage years, into my young adult years. In my process of freeing myself from held-on offenses, I had to deal with the root of what was going on. It was urgent because I knew that this cancer was more serious than the baggage that I held onto for years. **I was**

determined to fight, but I believed that holding onto those stressors were going to contribute to the growth of cancer that was in my breast. Stress is an aggressive monster, and it will not rest which is why self-care is important. My focus was to illuminate anything that could feed cancer and anything toxic; I had to get rid of it. I began my process by making phone calls, and I was intentional about it. The calls were uncomfortable to do but it was necessary. I was happy and relieved that I made the calls. The years of stress that I held onto were lifted from my shoulders during those moments.

I began to put myself first. I stopped worrying about everything else that was going wrong even within my family and carrying on the burdens of everyone else, which I did for many years. Two weeks after my diagnosis (July 2020), I decided to get rid of the offenses and negativity that I carried since childhood. My decision to do this was critical for my life.

Situations will come into your life that will make you look at life from a different perspective and through a different set of lenses. The challenges and tests that may come into your life, will cause you to look from a different perspective that is more significant and more impactful for your life's journey. In addressing my emotional, mental, and spiritual baggage, I began to feel lighter and more confident about my journey. I began to feel more responsible as I started to reclaim the years of hurt and lack; and now it was replaced with wholeness and joy, along with reminding myself that I am a priority. During this time, I discovered God's love for me in an entirely different way. I knew that when I discovered another layer of joy on this journey, I knew that was God saying that He was with me and that He's been with me since birth. It was designed that I was going to come out stronger than I did going in, because of how God was planning to use this journey as an encouragement for you. I was going to come out stronger in my faith than I've ever been. This was just the beginning of something new for me.

Surgery Day: October 28, 2020

The days leading up to my surgery were transformational. I had just moved into my new apartment, I had everything in order from my new bedroom set to my living room set. I pretty much had everything within 5-6 days of moving in. God provided me with the finances to purchase all that I needed for my new place. I couldn't sleep the night before my surgery. I believe I stayed up until 3 am and I had to be at the hospital no later than 8 am to prep for surgery. I cried the night before. I didn't cry because of fear. My tears were more so of anxiety because you never know what could happen. This was my first major surgery. Even in my tears, I knew that I was going to be OK. In your faith, you are going to have moments of apprehension. You're going to be a little concerned. But when you're walking forward in faith and simply have to do what you have to do and trust that God has your back, you always make it to the end of that chapter of your journey. On the day of my surgery, one of my best friend's Ashley accompanied me and sat for hours in the lobby during the surgery. By the grace of God, the surgery was successful with a slight medical emergency. During the surgical procedure, I had an allergic reaction to Ancef in which I did not know that I was allergic to. The surgeons mentioned that my mouth, tongue, and throat swelled and by the grace of God I am here. I had a successful surgery, and I also had the reconstruction procedure the same day. I did decide on a mastectomy of my right breast which had cancer. A mastectomy is the removal of the breast. The mastectomy was the best option for me because my cancer cells broke out of my milk duct and spread throughout my breast tissue. I was diagnosed with DCIS (Ductal Carcinoma in Situ), which is where my cancer cells were in my milk duct.

According to BreastCancer.org, DCIS is Ductal Carcinoma in Situ (DCIS) is non-invasive breast cancer. Ductal means that cancer starts inside the milk ducts, carcinoma refers to any cancer that begins in the skin or other tissues (including breast tissue) that cover or line the internal organs, and in situ means "in its original place". DCIS is called "non-invasive" because it hasn't spread beyond the milk duct into any normal surrounding breast tissue.

https://www.breastcancer.org/symptoms/types/dcis

In my case, my DCIS was discovered as invasive, and later discovered that the cancer cells broke out of my milk duct and spread throughout my right breast tissue, which is more of a reason why I am so glad that I decided to have a mastectomy. The discovery of cancer breaking out of my milk duct was found after my breast tissue was removed post-surgery.

Throughout the months, the cells eventually broke out of my milk duct and spread throughout my right breast tissue. Six of my lymph nodes were tested and they showed negative reports of cancer. What happens with a mastectomy? My entire right breast was removed, and people have asked me why I didn't get a double mastectomy. My desire and prayer is to become a mother one day, and I desire to breastfeed my child. I do believe that it is God's plan for me to one day become a mom and I'm trusting God with faith that my day will come. I have been proactive with having my exams and checking in with my doctor with any concerns that I may have with my left breast, just to be sure that everything is OK. As of April 2022, the cancer is still clear, and everything is well.

Life After Surgery

One may think at the age of now 33, with my mastectomy and having to take medication that could possibly create risk for me and having children and needing to make so many decisions that I didn't want to make at the age of 33. How do I cope? I had to think what mattered the most to me. I desired to live a life of abundant years of good health. I desire to be a wife and mother. I desire to continue to learn and discover me. I desire to complete my purpose that God has placed within me to do on this earth. I have so much to live for. Yes, I had to make some serious decisions at a young age. I still make life decisions each day regarding the medication that I take for the next four years. Making this decision every day is not easy. I have to make serious decisions at what I think is a young age; in the years when one is really entering a space of real adulthood. Years when I am honestly discovering myself as a woman. In the thirties, most people are either dating, married, building families, and/or growing in their lives. Who wants to have other thoughts, plans, and desires on hold because now you must focus on a life-threatening and altering health challenge in your youth or adult years; I wouldn't have before July 2020? If God told me that my journey consisted of cancer, I would've fought to avoid it. Why? Because I had other plans and hopes, but God had different plans for me during that time of my life. Even in our darkest moments of life, God will still allow you to illuminate and glow even amid your journey. Getting to the other side of that journey introduces you to strength and a fight that you never knew existed within you. There will come times within your life when you have to make serious decisions concerning your health. However, when you have to make these decisions, you have to do what you have to do so that you can live.

After my initial surgery (October 28, 2020), I had two additional surgeries (November 24th and December 18th). Due to cancer spreading through my breast tissue and preventive measures against cancer returning, my nipple was removed from my right breast. You may wonder if I feel insecure about my breast. You may ask, does she feel nervous that she will be judged by a male or significant other because she only has one breast? One thing that I do know is, my health is important to me. My breast has not changed or taken anything away from my femininity.

When you make a bold decision for your health, that is the most powerful thing that you could ever do, and it supersedes any physical change your body may go through. You could easily hide, run away, be fearful and let this thing control you. But because you have fought every storm, even the storm you're facing, or if you've watched someone else fight through their breast cancer journey and they've made the bold decision to live; that takes precedence over any image and possible insecurities. That in itself is strong. Everyone can't walk in that bold statement saying, "I can do anything" and "I'm determined to do anything to live and to live a life of abundance, no matter what". Any storm that you face head-on, represents the strength and the power of God in you. Nothing and no one can ever take that away from you. So, do I feel insecure? I can be honest; the thought came to my mind. But then I had to remember, why I made my decision and how powerful it was because my life depended on it. I made a decision that saved my life. I am stronger as a woman than I have ever been. I am bolder and more confident than I've ever been. This journey will change your life! I have decided to live my life joyfully in wholeness and peace, along with putting myself first. I decided to trust God, even while facing a storm that I'd never experienced before. I learned to walk by faith and not by sight. Many people didn't catch their cancer early or live years beyond what others may have hoped for. However, their journeys and lives lived on in those whom they touched and inspired. God allowed me to live through these times for a purpose and I will live it out loud. God has given me a voice and boldness to provide hope to others and the families of those who are supporting a loved one on their journey. I would like to share this with you, know that anything with God is possible. There's a purpose in His will and in everything that He guides us through. Sometimes moments occur within our lives in which we may not understand why. I know because I too lived it. When I felt my lowest during my first week, I had to get on my knees, humble myself and open myself to receive the love, comfort, strength, joy, and endurance of

God. During this time, I remained in prayer and the presence of God. I had to discover how He saw me. He sees me as His daughter, as His beloved. My go-to scripture that kept me grounded in my relationship with God is Proverbs 3:5-6 "Trust in the Lord with all thine heart; and lean not unto thine own understanding. In all thy ways acknowledge Him, and He shall direct thy paths."

This scripture kept me strengthened and focused during some of the most challenging moments in my life, and I pray that if you have your scripture that you continuously MEDITATE on it. If you don't have a scripture that you lean on, take Proverbs 3:5-6 and apply it to your life as well as your perception while moving forward. The first scripture that I focused in on and applied to my life when I gave my life to Christ was Proverbs 3:5-6. I did not know that this scripture was going to help me through every storm that I faced in life. That scripture is the foundational for my life. I pray that this same scripture brings a blessing and hope to you as well.

Life as a Single Woman, Post Surgery

The week when I received my diagnosis, it was extremely hard. I began to think about how my life would change for family, relationships, and all the dreams and desires that I have for my life. I began to think about how this diagnosis will bring a shift or a change in my life. However, during the time I had support. I had positive people around me, who encouraged me throughout the way. Nonetheless, there was this thought about whether or not I will be able to have children, and if this cancer would limit my chances of having children.

The thought of someone not accepting me didn't come to mind, because I was blessed to have a significant friend who was there by my side during this time. However, things began to shift and change within our friendship. Regardless of why our connection while dating shifted, I am grateful for my friend. How we engaged each other changed, and I believe that it did not necessarily have to do with my diagnosis. I know from the person directly that the pursuit was no longer there. Only God knows if that was the truth or if it had anything else to do with cancer. Only God knows. However, I was later faced with a conversation that I wasn't prepared to have. I began to reconnect with a former friend of mine, whom I dated years ago; and this was after my mastectomy. A few weeks into our reconnecting, I asked him a question that was important to me. I asked him if he would accept me knowing that I've had a mastectomy and replacement with an implant, and at this point, my nipple was removed. He followed with a text, "I would have to see what it looks like" and I followed through and said, "Thank you for your honesty and I respect what you texted. However, I am comfortable in how I look and how I feel like a woman, but I get that I come with a package." My package to me included a missing nipple. He then recanted his statement and he said he used a bad choice of words. But even in his response, whether he said he used a bad choice of words and it wasn't his intention, the reality set in for me at that moment. I had to then accept that I am a little slightly different now, and I am prepared and ok knowing that there are going to be conversations that I'm going to have to have with whomever I date. To add, he and I never reconnected romantically. I will be OK with their response. I am ok with a guy possibly having a problem or concern with my diagnosis and fears of it returning. Having cancer is a major experience that you have to make mature decisions for the sake of your life. Matters are going to arise in relationships where a person may feel that they can't mentally emotionally, or spiritually support you and it's OK. When I had this conversation with this gentleman, it made me realize that this is the journey on the road that

I'm going forward. I had to check myself and my emotional and mental gage to be secure in me. I had to also be honest with my feelings when moments or thoughts like this would occur. I know that they are going to be times when someone may not want to be with me because of my surgery. But one thing that I love that God has done within me through this journey is knowing and remembering how much He loves me as His daughter. That may sound very cliché right. But it's the truth, this is coming from someone that was neglected emotionally and who lived a life feeling that they weren't good enough to be loved by anyone even by God Himself. So, when God took me in as His daughter, it revealed to me who He was as my Father. I began to love on myself and see myself as a person who deserved to be loved. Knowing and understanding who you are in God will help you to love yourself. He will begin to help you to love yourself beyond the looks, but also the strength and the power that you have within yourself. That is priceless and significantly more impactful for your life than you know. I'm saying all of this to say that, you are beautiful.

If you are single love on you. If you are supporting a friend or significant other, love on them and be present. If you are single, there is someone who is going to be so excited about you. They will be blown away and crazily in love with you, no matter what you have, because they are the ones who God chose for you. They are going to be the ones who will be present and blown away in love with you. With God, because you two will share regarding God's love and compassion, the intentions and purpose of you two meeting will be established and bloom within the relationship. Being single within this is a journey, it is not one to be fearful of. Trust that if God brought you this far, and if He's using you as a voice and as a testimony of His love even within your family. Trust in Him and do what He desires you to do during this time. He will grant you the desires of your heart and more. God will give you the desires that He wants for you, and you must trust Him. Trust and believe that everything is in sync with what you've laid before Him. You are beautiful and loved. If anyone decides not to be with you because of your physical appearance, they are not the one for you. You deserve someone who honors God, and who you are to God as His child. You are a warrior. Facing cancer and receiving the diagnosis is not something that an average person without faith and strength can receive and grow from. Understand that you are worth more than you may even know, and even if you do know your worth, continue to embrace the comfort of God and walk in it. You are fearfully and wonderfully made in the eyesight and image of God.

Journal Entries:

Pre-Biopsy Journal 6/13/20 10:32 pm

Last week I went in for a mammogram, after my doctor ordered it about three weeks ago. I went in for a lump in my left breast, only to discover that I needed a biopsy within my right breast. After the mammogram appointment, I was calm and surprised that I wasn't panicking and concerned.

Today on 6/13, I cried with the thoughts about the biopsy which is scheduled to happen in a few weeks. I am worried and anxious, which are emotions that I hadn't felt at all since receiving the news that I needed to have a mammogram. Thankfully when I had my moment today, I was surrounded with love, a breast cancer survivor and the two women, who were divinely placed near me prayed with me. I returned to my car and began to think, Lord even though I haven't had my biopsy I did think Lord

I'm 32.... then I began to think maybe this is a punishment from God for not moving and completing goals and visions that He trusted me with, or for any disobedience that I lived with in my life. I thought any and everything.

At that very moment, I remembered that I planned to call one of my spiritual advisors. I called her and we talked about everything and caught up with each other since we haven't talked in months. Before ending the call, I told her about my appointment and unbeknownst to me she was diagnosed in December 24, 2019, and it was an early detection. The doctors were able to remove the cancer, and also reconstruct her breasts. It was not an accident that we talked, and our phone conversation was a total of six and a half hours long.

Before we said our good-byes, she told me that the Lord has plans for me and He did not bring me this far just to leave me and to make this the ending of my life. It was like I needed to hear that word from the Lord. After we got off the phone, the Holy Spirit led me to play "Loved by You" by Travis Green. The Lord knows and sees me, and I'm still loved. This experience with the biopsy is a test of my faith and a test to add to my testimony. I told someone earlier that my life is a testimony. A testimony of God's love, protection, grace, covering, and intentions. God is not done with me, I believe it for you as well. Regardless of how things look, God is not done. Through your story, you and others who need encouragement will see the handprint of God. You are loved; and in the chaos, the Lord is our joy. I'm ok and I will be no matter what the results may be after my biopsy, on June 25th. You are loved and so am I.

Journal Entry

June 12, 2020

Psalm 51:1-19 NKJV

"Have mercy upon me, O God, According to Your lovingkindness; According to the multitude of Your tender mercies, Blot out my transgressions. Wash me thoroughly from my iniquity, And cleanse me from my sin. For I acknowledge my transgressions, and my sin is always before me. Against You, You only, have I sinned, And done this evil in Your sight— That You may be found just when You speak, And blameless when You judge. Behold, I was brought forth in iniquity, And in sin, my mother conceived me. Behold, you desire truth in the inward parts, and in the hidden part, You will make me to know wisdom. Purge me with hyssop, and I shall be clean; Wash me, and I shall be whiter than snow. Make me hear joy and gladness, That the bones You have broken may rejoice. Hide Your face from my sins, And blot out all my iniquities. Create in me a clean heart, O God, And renew a steadfast spirit within me. Do not cast me away from Your presence, And do not take Your Holy Spirit from me. Restore to me the joy of Your salvation, And uphold me by Your generous Spirit. Then I will teach transgressors Your ways, And sinners shall be converted to You. Deliver me from the guilt of bloodshed, O God, The God of my salvation, And my tongue shall sing aloud of Your righteousness. O Lord, open my lips, And my mouth shall show forth Your praise. For You do not desire sacrifice, or else I would give it; You do not delight in burnt offering. The sacrifices of God are a broken spirit, A broken and a contrite heart— These, O God, You will not despise. Do good in Your good pleasure to Zion; Build the walls of Jerusalem. Then You shall be pleased with the sacrifices of righteousness, With burnt offering and whole burnt offering; Then they shall offer bulls on Your altar."

November 4, 2020: Post Surgery

No pain

Drains are becoming less and less. I believe that our blessing matches our faith. We cannot pick and choose what we believe God to do. It's either, you are all in or out.

Faith keeps us balanced and leveled.

Any road that leads to a powerful victorious end, is difficult and it takes intentional work, fearless and wavering faith, strength, and commitment.

Every experience on the journey, God has favored and graced me to keep moving, even when I feel that I can't.

I will continue to press forward. I am victorious! When I make it over (because I will) I will share the story.

God, You have made me strong, resilient, and determined. I've been through so much in life that I had no choice but to fight this and win. Accepting fear and remaining in any kind of sadness I am certain that I wouldn't even be where I am.

I had my tears and low moments the first week or two and a few afterward. Some people didn't understand why the cancer entered my life and almost caused added stress to my day. However, I am thankful that I had the boldness had to kindly remove myself and focus on what I knew You desired for me.

That's the only reason why I am in the place I'm in now. I will see this through. I'm good though; sincerely and humbly. I give God all the glory for this, because I wouldn't have made it on my own. God placed people around me closely, who held me up and was strong enough to do so. This isn't an easy bag to carry, but I took on the journey and walked. God made my faith and strength stronger than I ever thought it would be.

November 11, 2020 10:25 am

Encouragement

Glory to God! God knows everything and He has a plan to help us navigate through any and every moment in our lives. Let God be God (protector, teacher, provider, peace....) even when times feel rough. Allow Him full access to cultivate and build your faith; and prepare you to receive the blessing and newness that's on the other side.

The person I was when I first received my diagnosis, went through an entire transformation. The person I was in July 2020 is not the same person I am today. I thank God for the newness of faith, strength, power, and wisdom. Let God be God and watch.

Prayer Changes Everything

When facing a cancer diagnosis, you must be aware that this is a very serious and life-changing situation, but it is so important not to dwell on the negative throughout your journey. Surround yourself with faith-driven people and people who are filled with wisdom, and my prayer is that they are filled with godly wisdom. It is so important to be aware of who you allow around you during these times, so that you can successfully and victoriously conquer this this journey and all that comes with it. The times faced are so precious and delicate that if you allow the wrong person in your ear, they may stress you and cause you to feel defeated when fighting is your option of choice. Walking BY Faith is your choice not fear.

You cannot allow any and everybody in your ear, because they can give you false information or false advice. Some people may possibly make your situation worse, and it will be outside of God's will for you (for this particular time). There are a lot of people that I did not tell when I first received my diagnosis because I understood how important and how serious this experience was going to be for me. I did not need the naysayers, the doubters, the folks filled with anxiety and just paranoia. You have to pray and ask God for discernment. The first week of receiving the diagnosis was not the easiest for me; it wasn't, and I had to lay before God and pray and cry. I had to be honest about how I felt. I had to tell God that I was afraid, that I was concerned, that I was even upset with Him. I told God that I went through so much in my life and was now facing this diagnosis.

I asked God when will my battles come to an end. I wanted to live and be happy for a change in my life. I was tired. People may think that being mad with God or upset with God is a bad thing, but it's not. You must be intentional about your truth; you must be transparent with God. Honesty is key to breaking through every fear. When you are transparent during your alone time with God and tell Him that you are upset and why. As you process through everything, admit that you feel heartbroken. Speak in honesty and truth. God cannot break through what you are not honest about. God cannot prepare you to rise in victory when you are not honest in your weakness. God cannot show you His truth when you are not upfront about what you don't believe or what you don't have the assurance that He will fulfill. Tell the truth. It's one thing when a person just doesn't care, but it's another thing when you're like, God I just don't believe, so please help me with my unbelief. Help me. God will give you peace, hope, and the wisdom you need to make it through this moment of your life. God will increase and expand your belief in Him, but you must be honest. When you think about a natural parent, most parents will tell their child if you don't like something or if you feel concerned about something, ask questions and talk to me so that I'll know. This is no different from God. God desires for us to come to Him, to ask Him questions, to be upfront and honest so that He can help us. God knows what we lack with our faith in Him. He is not ashamed or offended. God knows the areas within us where we lack belief. Therefore, we have to speak it so that we can own where our faith is at the time and prepare to be strengthened in the areas presented before God. He desires for us to speak it and not live fake fantasy life like everything is ok. We have to speak HOPE even when our faith is shaken, for it to become a reality for us. Sometimes you have to hear your fears be spoken out of your mouth for you to realize, "Wow, this is for real? I don't believe this, I have a challenge with my faith.". A lot of people suppress worries when they are afraid of living in their truth or speaking the truth. Sometimes the truth is I know I'm afraid, but I'll mask it because I don't want to appear as being weak. That's not how God desires for us to operate with Him. He desires for us to speak the truth to Him, especially in our weakest moments. He desires us to walk in truth and He desires for us to receive the truth of what He has for our lives.

During the first week of my diagnosis, I spent so much time with God. I had a prayer partner, who prayed with me for an hour every single day during the early stages of my diagnosis; because I knew God, prayer and counseling was going to get me through this. I knew that it was a very serious and very fragile moment for me. Retreating to the "comfort" and familiarity of depression could have been detrimental for me. I was a person who battled with depression for so long and honestly felt unhappy and comfortable in it. So, if this diagnosis was presented to a person, who is known to have battled with depression from childhood up until adult years, you would think the diagnosis report would be a trigger that would place the person at their breaking point or not wanting to exist. However, God had me at that moment and I'm grateful.

Prayer changes things. As a praying community of a few people, I knew who were solid in their faith and they were on board and most importantly, they understood and knew what God was doing through my life: even through the diagnosis. You must be intentional in your decision making during this time, and that includes facing any challenge within your life. You cannot tell everybody everything and you must understand, that there's a time and a season that certain people need to know certain things. Everybody does not need to know everything when you are going through your challenges. Some people mean well, and some people simply do not mean well at all, and they will try to either scare you or try to take you off course. Some people will even try to do whatever they can to dishearten you, because they want you to live in depression or hurt. It feels weird to think there are people in this time and day who wish bad on others, but there are. So, I leave you with this, be prayerful about everything in your journey. People have come up to me in my doctor's office and were amazed at how God kept me during this journey. The doctors were even inspired by my attitude and determination during this process. Some people heard about my testimony or whom I've spoken to about my journey, and they would say, "Wow Tee, I had no idea that you were going through that." God has a way of taking us through valley moments. As we are in prayer and in His presence, we will not look like what we're going through or even came out of. Does that indicate that you are falsifying your peace? This assures that God is keeping you through it so intentionally, comforting you and providing strength that you will not look like what you're going through. You don't have to look like what you're going through. During this time, I was intentional about finding my joy. As I mentioned previously in this chapter, I was a child that went through depression for many years. I was going through battles back-to-back that when this came, I felt like "God, when will this stop?" So, when I learned that the cause of my cancer could've very well been because of underlying stress and depression that I suppressed for so many years, I was intentional about living my life. I had yet to allow myself to live a life of joy and intentional joy regardless of how that was going to look. I had to remove stressors, I had to remove things that were weighing on me. I had to be deliberate about removing myself from certain situations and conversations. I had to understand what boundaries meant, what it looks like, and what I desired of it. When I understood what boundaries meant, I was able to keep my joy and peace as a priority. Whatever it took for me to do that, I did it.

I prayed and asked God to show me how to navigate through this journey. I told God that I desire to be happy, and I wanted to live a life that I've always prayed for. God also removed me from an environment that kept me bound in so much emotional, spiritual, and mental despair that included emptiness in me, that He blessed me with a new location and my place. I made it my own and I love it. I was approved for my apartment after a few days of applying, and I said to God this is Your plan and purpose for my life. My approval was processed three weeks before my surgery. God didn't even stop there, He even showed me favor on my job. He showed me favor with the team that He blessed me with at the hospital. God also showed me favor throughout my journey with correcting and removing breast cancer. God has done exceeding abundantly above all that I could've asked or thought of. I was intentional in my prayers and by Walking By Faith, it caused me to see beyond my situation at the time.

I titled this chapter *Prayer Changes Everything* because prayer changed and saved my life throughout this time from my diagnosis in July, up until December. God has given me the love, joy, peace, comfort, and clarity that I have prayed for so many years. He moved into my life instantly, well what I felt was instant. There were years that I prayed and hoped for a change to come. I had to go through the valley of being prepared, to be able to humbly receive care and honor the blessings that He had for me. I had no idea that in 2020, during the pandemic that my life would change completely.

Prayer sustains you. Prayer centers you. Prayer will lead and keep you solid on the foundation of faith that you have. Prayer is your intimacy with God and even when you don't know what to say, God can move and place blessings in your path that will keep you sustained. Divine Interception.

I had two choices: to fight or flight. In the beginning of my journey, even when I had a small thought of taking flight, faith and determination kept me. My thought of flight could've been the fact that I was nervous about dying. During the first week I didn't have an immediate thought about dying, but I just felt that my hopes and desires were going to die. I thought the prayers that I've prayed and placed before God were going to die. I didn't think that I was going to physically die. I thought that everything that I hoped for was no longer going to exist. But God is faithful, and He was able to comfort me because I was honest with Him. If there's anything that you take from this chapter, I pray that you take the understanding and the importance of being honest and truthful before God seriously. God desires for us to be real with ourselves and with Him. As I've mentioned He knows everything, but He wants us to speak the truth so that He can reveal His truth to us for us to move forward. I love you.

Breast Cancer Information

Breast Cancer affects one in eight women during their lives. No one knows why some women get breast cancer, but there are many risk factors. Risks that you cannot change include:

- Age - the risk rises as you get older
- Genes - two genes, BRCA1 and BRCA2, greatly increase the risk. Women who have family members with breast or ovarian cancer may wish to be tested for the genes.
- Personal Factors - beginning periods before age 12 or going through menopause after age 55

Other risks include obesity, using hormone replacement therapy (also called menopausal hormone therapy), taking birth control pills, drinking alcohol, not having children or having your first child after age 35, and having dense breasts.

Symptoms of breast cancer may include a lump in the breast, a change in size or shape of the breast, and discharge from a nipple. Breast self-exams and mammography can help find breast cancer early, when it is most treatable. One possible treatment is surgery. It could be a lumpectomy or a mastectomy. Other treatments include radiation therapy, chemotherapy, hormone therapy, and targeted therapy. Targeted therapy uses drugs or other substances that attack cancer cells with less harm to normal cells. Men can have breast cancer, too, but it is rare.

Fasting and eating healthy support your recovery and healing for surgery and treatment. I also learned that dates are good for natural sugar. A diet of abstaining from sugar, meat (some baked fish is ok), sodas, and liquor is greatly beneficial during your journey.

This Was Not a Mistake

This journey is not by mistake. There were many times that I wondered why. I thought, how can a healthy person who may have had 3 or 4 common colds throughout the years and never been hospitalized have to face this? I believe battling with depression since childhood weighed heavy on me. I may not have felt the stress physically, but internally something was going on that I was aware of. Medicine can say how cancer occurs, but what I do believe in my case is the undetected stress that I endured over so many years, and then later on in my 20s detected and diagnosed as major depression affected me internally. Per genetic test, the breast cancer that I had, or any breast cancer was not directly genetically linked to me. I believe by the grace of God, the cancer ended with me. I'm thankful that God allowed this diagnosis to be discovered at such an early stage. I mentioned earlier in this book that when the technicians pulled the samples from my breast, they said this was the earliest catch they've ever seen. God planned that the cancer is discovered at a period that it was. And I'm thankful to God that I not only survived this stage of my journey, but I'm a survivor for all those who will have their own. But I want to encourage you to remember that what you internalize, will become what you take on throughout your days. What you carry will become a part of you. You have to remember that your life, your wellness, your body, your spirit, and your heart are important. If there's anyone in this world who understands that it must be you. It's okay if other people may not understand it, but you need to. You are valuable, you are precious, you are needed, and you were born with a purpose. Your purpose was not to live a life of depression, stress, illness, and pain but a life full of abundance, purpose, and joyful experiences in between. After all the things that

I've experienced in my life, even leading up to my cancer diagnosis, I can say, *Lord, I keep taking hits after hits after the hits, but what I know now is that You have me.* He has you too. God allows each of us to see life in another way than we have ever experienced before. He allowed me to experience a faith that I never thought I would experience before, and this is just part of my journey and story. I am just thankful and humbly grateful that I lived through this to be a blessing of hope and encouragement for you. Sharing and believing God's plan for your life of prosperity and purpose brought joy to my heart and I pray that it does the same for you. Because of my assignment to you, you encouraged me and helped me to finish this book. Never forget who your Divine Interceptor is and know that He has your future, destiny, purpose, choices, calling, and power all in His hands. Victory is won therefore, continue to Walk BY Faith, celebrate each victory (regardless of the size) during your journey and allow God to give you all that you need. God's blessings to you.

I love you, Taneya.

Walk By Faith:

21 Days of Empowerment

As I was preparing this portion of the book, I asked God to lead me through this writing to give you a timely message of hope and encouragement during these 21 days. Twenty-One days represents change. Not only can the change be made within you physically, but also spiritually. My prayer for you is that your faith is developed to mirror where you desire to be and grow throughout your journey. No one ever mentioned that change feels pleasant, but what I know is there's a purpose to every journey that you embark upon. Walk into your day commanding peace, love, clarity, and wholeness to consume your day. As written in Job 38:12, "Have you ever commanded the morning to appear and caused the dawn to rise in the east?" Walk into your day knowing that God is in total control and that He did not allow anything to happen to you that He wasn't aware of. Everything that we experience in life has a purpose.

My prayer for us on this journey: *Father, I am joining together with Your beloved, declaring that this is the day that You have made. The rejoicing of our hearts and adoration of who You are will be lifted high today, regardless of what the day holds. Father, bless Your beloved with a peace that surpasses all understanding and awaken the joy that You have placed within them from the day they were born. I pray that the strength of Your power, will lead them throughout the day. I pray that their strength will be renewed, they will mount up with wings like eagles, run and not be weary and walk and not fear as declared in Isaiah 40:31. Give Your beloved a renewed strength that is built only because of Your joy. We love You, Lord. We know that Your timing and all that we have encountered is not in vain. We love You and thank You in JESUS' name, AMEN!*

<u>Declaration:</u> The timing of the Lord makes me stronger and wiser. I am victorious in this Faith Building.

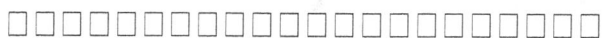

Day 1: Following and Applying Instructions

**Which is easier, to say, 'Your sins are forgiven you,' or to say, 'Rise up and walk'? But that you may know that the Son of Man has power on earth to forgive sins – He said to the man who was paralyzed, 'I say to you, arise, take up your bed, and go to your house'. ~Luke 5:23-24 NKJV**

Receiving instructions is the easy part for some of us. Taking the instructions to apply to our lives is where the challenges are revealed. Today will be filled with moments where you will have to make decisions that may feel intimidating. If you are or have been anything like me, trying to move in your own will and strength, it will always place you at a roadblock or with your back against the wall. When your back is against the wall, the only direction you can go is forward. My challenge to you today is to move forward. The pressure may feel heavy, but I need you to walk forward. It is easy for the doctors to say you have an illness, but hearing "Here are the treatments and surgeries you have to do to save your life" is hard. It is easy to listen to the plans and instructions of the doctors, but the challenging yet most powerful thing to do is, rise and walk; even when anxiety or fear tries to creep in. When you rise up, you are determined to get up and fight. The paralyzed man at the pool of Bethesda did not allow his current condition to weigh him down any longer. He applied his faith to the instructions given and walked into his healing. The healing of your walk isn't just physically, but it's also spiritually. As you're moving forward, process all that the day holds and know that God is with you each step that you take. God has you in the palm of His hand.

Day 2: Happiness is a Priority for you.

Happy is that people, that is in such a case: yea, happy is that people, whose God is the Lord. ~Psalm 144:15 KJV

What have you done for yourself lately that brought you happiness for the day? Joy is an entirely different level of existing and a gift that no one can take from you. Joy is internal and lasts for an eternity. However, let's talk about happiness. Happiness is a temporary experience that you can do within a day for yourself or something that someone may be able provide for you. My question for you is: When was the last time that you did something that made you happy? What I love about happiness is that you have control over it. So, anything that has been a stressor for you that is outside of your process throughout this journey, I challenge you today to discover a way to unplug from it.

Factors that can dampen your happiness can be a bothersome bill or a car that may give you headaches with the issues that it can bring. You may feel that it may be time to get a new car (my testimony). Your happiness can be discovering a hobby that you never took the time to experience, taking a walk, and committing to enjoying the moments daily or every other day. Your piece of happiness can be as deep as resolving a long-lasting feud or disagreement with a person. It can be going out and grabbing a jumbo slice of pizza or taking a ride in your car with the windows down with the music playing at the volume of your choice. Discover what brings you happiness and make that a top priority for today and practice that same decision and mindset throughout this week. Again, what have you done lately that brings you happiness? This journey is a process. However, I challenge you today to not only take care of your health and make it top priority, but also understand that discovering happiness is a part of this process as well. Happiness is not something to be neglected, you deserve to be happy even though everything around you is telling you to feel otherwise. From experience, happiness allows your healing process to become more effective. Practice your daily routines of embracing joy and finding your happiness in every day. YOU CAN DO THIS!

Day 3: Who is in your space?

He that walketh with wise men shall be wise: but a companion of fools shall be destroyed. ~Proverbs 13:20 KJV

Today, I want you to be cognizant of who's in your space. Most times when facing challenges in life, people will say, never face or fix your challenge alone; which is accurate. However, it is important to be aware of who you have in your personal space daily. You are in a time where you need someone or people who are encouraging, gentle, wise, and invested in learning and understanding your condition. Family, friends, and associates may mean well. However, not all company is healthy company during your journey. As you go throughout your day today, realize that you have the right to assess who to include in your daily life or those whom you may need to limit having close access to you daily. A person having direct access to you is not just physically, but also mentally and spiritually. You have the right to pay attention to the language, behaviors, and reactions of those individuals during this journey; and remove some as you feel needed. Any level of ignorance and lack of spiritual maturity one may have, can affect how you view your illness and how you approach moments that may shake your faith. This is a time where you put your space, time, and those to whom you give access to your life during this moment at top priority. You must be intentional about knowing who to have in your space (spiritually, mentally, and emotionally). The current times are delicate, and your well-being is important. Understand that you have the right to decide on what you disclose regarding information, personal feelings, and certain truths of how you're processing through this journey with people. Everyone is not privy to every moment during this time of your life. Making this decision does not mean that they're toxic individuals. This decision means that you realize or understand how important this time of your life is. During this time, you need people who are adding and not subtracting from your life; people who are cultivating and not demolishing your life. Pay attention to who comes into your space today.

Day 4: I am yours and you are mine

Do not be afraid, for I have ransomed you. I have called you by name; you are mine. ~Isaiah 43:1b NLT

Do you know that God has claimed you as His own? He is happy that He made you from His own hands. Do you know that God is so in love with you and reminds you each day that you are His? Breath shows there's still a purpose for you being here. A heartbeat means that there is still more life for you to live. A mind that functions and recognizes God as a Father, means there is still life in the connection of knowing who God is in you. God said that I am yours and you are mine. God will not allow anything to happen to His children without there being a purpose within it. God said that you are Mine. You do not belong to this illness. You are not in bondage of the treatment and diagnosis. You are a child of God, with a process that everyone may not understand. Sometimes we don't understand some life experiences, but in our lack of understanding comes a time of surrendering to understand.

Today, remember that you belong to our Father in heaven, who knows every moment of your life. You are not a victim nor a servant of the illness. You are a victor and master through the power of Jesus over an illness. Jesus made you new, whole, and powerful over every illness and disease. Regardless of what comes throughout this day, know who you can call on, and who lives on the inside of you. You are God's child whom He loves more than you'll ever truly know.

Day 5: Time with God

Seek the Lord and his strength, seek his face continually.

~1 Chronicles 16:11 KJV

The timing of God is strategic and intentional. As God is time and the Creator, there are moments and situations set in place to help you learn and experience God like you never have before. What does that mean? Have you ever noticed moments when you just do things out of habit? There's not a major reason or purpose to why you do it, it's just a habit? For example, most times people pray and read devotions out of habit. Some do it and allow the words to mediate, whereas others do it and it doesn't have any effect on them. God doesn't want His children to just come to Him due to a programed habit. God desires us to come to Him daily and with the intentions of being close with

Him. During any adverse moment, there are so many questions like, "God, why me?" My prayer for you today is that you ask God, what are You trying to show me and develop within me? The enemy plans to steal, kill and destroy. To steal your promise, kill your faith, and destroy your destiny. WE ARE NOT GIVING HIM SPACE OR TIME TO DO THAT AT ALL!!!

Timing. How does timing relate to facing the journey of breast cancer? There are times when God will allow His chosen ones to carry out a message that He is still in control. The strength, determination, and peace that He provides His children during these times are only from Him. Faith takes growth and development; and without faith being stretched, who would we be as people. When the timing of God requires a level of faith to be developed, count it all joy. James 1:2 says, "Count it all joy." When things look contrary to what you desire or believe, trust God and seek the joy of the Lord within you. The joy of the Lord is your strength. Joy doesn't always mean that you are jumping up and down or skipping down the street all the time. Joy is an internal peace that no one or nothing can remove. Joy is your place of being. Joy is a mentality and lifestyle rather than an emotion. Your joy is internal, and my prayer is that it is awakened even during a moment of sadness today. The timing of the Lord is purposeful. Joy is foundational and will keep you standing, even when you want to break. Remember, the joy of the Lord is your strength.

Day 6: Spirit, lead me where my trust is without borders.

'Lord, help!' they cried in their trouble, and he saved them from their distress. He calmed the storm to a whisper and stilled the waves. ~Psalm 107:28-29 NLT

Borders are made to separate. Receiving any diagnosis that has tested your faith, belief, and reality of life has the potential to cause walls to form. Hesitation, uncertainty, and fear are expected in adverse situation, and it is normal. However, in the building of every wall it will eventually come down. What will cause the borders to fall? A fearless mind and clear perception does not happen overnight. In fact, after many days of kicking, screaming, crying, questioning, and more, the process of breaking down barriers and walls that shatters your faith will take place. Do you know that God made your mind, and because you are of God, what you tell your mind to do, it will do? If you are in a space of fear and depression, and you are determined to overcome it, you will. Your mind is a servant to you and not a lord over you. The matters of life will always challenge our understanding of how powerful we are in our thoughts. God's word says in Proverbs 23:7, "For as he thinks in his heart so is he...." God knows the fear, anxiety, and worry. He knows every concern that you have. God will cultivate your faith as you trust in Him during this time.

Today is a day to acknowledge the levels of trust you have with God and to be honest about it. Praying in honesty with God during this time will be the greatest decision you can choose. Believe it or not, if you are in doubt about your trust in God, your trust kicked in the very moment you were made aware of your diagnosis. Your trust was established the moment you began to read this book. Your trust kicked in when you decided to report to your first appointment, because you were determined to take action. God is a loving Father, and He will give you the wisdom and comfort you need to walk through this process. My prayer today is that you trust God to mold you wherever your faith is unsure and that you begin the process of living in freedom and peace while discovering it daily. Be gentle with yourself, because every level you enter in this process will require a refined faith of you. The border will come down and even as you move forward and walk in faith, there will be times when the borders will arise again, but you will be prepared to break them down. You will see the purpose and plans of God even when they try to arise. Each day that you are determined to live, the stronger you will become.

Day 7: No Stressing today. "I will not complain today."

Then Jesus said, "Come to me, all of you who are weary and carry heavy burdens, and I will give you rest. ~Matthew 11:28 NLT

Stress. Stress has a purpose and it deals with challenges the way it desires to. My prayer for you today is that you realize how significant your life, your health, and your future is. My prayer is that you look at the many blessings you have. Whatever comes your way today that may ruffle your feathers, I want you to filter it through the mindset and lens of being victorious. We are only as victorious daily as we make our minds to be. The Bible says that we are to take on the mind of Christ daily. Christ went through many challenges in life, but instead of running from every odd and testing moment sent against Him, He faced what He had to and His weapon was prayer. Communication with God is the tool I had to use. In times of fear or uncertainty, prayer kept me in a place that was a safety zone for me. So, my prayer today is that you use the wisdom of God with prayer, that you have to overcome any challenge that comes your way today. Stress is not your portion today. Peace, joy, love, and resiliency are your portion. Set a limit on how much pressure/stress you will allow to be a part of your life today. Trials are going to come which is inevitable. Depression will not control your day. Anxiety will not control your day. You are victorious! You are strong! You are powerful! Your testimony of resiliency and strength will carry you through this journey.

Day 8: Breathe and Release

For I know the thoughts that I think toward you, saith the Lord, thoughts of peace, and not of evil, to give you an expected end.

~Jeremiah 29:11 KJV

Simple exercises of self-care moments that appear to be so easy and small to accomplish are some of the most neglected. Here's my charge to you today: Stop, Inhale, Exhale, and Release. You deserve to embrace and take moments to stop, inhale, exhale, and release daily. Sending Peace, Love, and Joy to you.

Day 9: Time.

But you must not forget this one thing, dear friends: A day is like a thousand years to the Lord, and a thousand years is like a day.[9] The Lord isn't really being slow about his promise, as some people think. No, he is being patient for your sake. He does not want anyone to be destroyed, but wants everyone to repent.

~2 Peter 3:8-9 NLT

When I think about time, I think about life experiences. How do life experiences impact and shape us? What happens to us during that time as we are being stretched to another level of faith and strength, that we never knew existed within us? Throughout my journey, I began to see and understand that time was and is a gift. What we do with time expresses our appreciation of the gift of time. The word of God speaks that there is a time for everything in Ephesians. During this journey, I am praying that you realize and understand that you have the right to express how you feel at any time during this journey. Each moment that you express your emotions, joys, fears, concerns, and worries are all acceptable. There's nothing abnormal about how you feel during the times that you have to face. Each second and minute you remain authentic to how you feel will develop strength in this fight. Regardless of any burdensome moments you encounter, remember that time is a gift to you. God will not allow anything to happen in your timing that He has not already prepared you to overcome. Without time, we will never know who we are. Without time, you would never know how strong you are. Without time, you would never know your purpose. Always remember that you have a purpose. The purpose is expressed and revealed in time, so just take a moment to realize how precious time is and enjoy your day. Take time out for yourself. As I mentioned, time is a gift and you deserve to receive the greatest gift in it. This is not a time of defeat nor a time of disaster. This is a time of triumph, victory, and strength. God placed you on this earth. You were formed and molded in His divine time with a purpose. Be blessed and know that you are cherished.

Day 10: Victorious

For the LORD your God is going with you! He will fight for you against your enemies, and he will give you victory! ~Deuteronomy 20:4 NLT

As I'm writing this day of encouragement for you, and after the Lord gave me the title for this day which is "Victorious", the song by Donnie McClurkin *Victorious* settled in my heart. The specific verse that played through my mind was, "We are victorious, we are victorious. Nothing can conquer us, we are victorious." What I believe is God's purpose for you was and remains for you to be victorious. It was already established before you entered this journey of your life. However, when challenges come our way, most times we can get into a space of thinking they were defeated because we think, "God, why would you bring this into my life?" Victorious doesn't always mean that you're going to feel strong, that you're going to feel like a winner, that everything around you is peaches and cream, or everything is filled with sunshine and rainbows. Just because there's a little gray in your day, the storms are crashing, or the waves feel like they are sinking you, does not mean that you're not victorious. I believe a victorious person is someone who faces the storm, by hopping in the boat and moving as the waves come. Victorious to me is a person finding a way to survive no matter what they have to do, because they are determined to survive. In moments like this, there will be times when you may not see the sunshine every day or in each moment. However, due to the resiliency of a person, they will face the storm head on. As you weather the storm, the sunshine will come and that same victorious spirit that you had in the storm will live the time when the sun comes out. You are victorious in the good and bad times. You are victorious in each stage that this journey takes you, whether you are going through treatment or in recovery. Whether you received your diagnosis for the first time, pre-surgery or post-surgery. Whether you recently received a diagnosis, and you must face this journey head-on, you are victorious. A victorious person is determined to face the storm, and receive the strength, faith, and purpose within them to push forward. One who is not afraid or unapologetic about how they are going to pursue the purpose in everything that their life brings. You are victorious no matter what stage you are in during this journey.

Day 11: It is ok to feel tired emotionally and mentally, but I don't want you to get stuck there.

And we know that all things work together for good to them that love God, to them who are the called according to his purpose.

~Romans 8:28 KJV

    In June 2021, I experienced a great loss, one of the greatest Women of God, who God has ever placed in my life. To experience grief at that level was heavy on me, and the week following her death was just as difficult (spiritually, mentally, and emotionally). On top of facing her death, I was in the planning stages of my _Cherish The Steps_ event. Two weeks later, I decided to call my friend who's more like a mother figure to me to set up a time for us to take our weekly walk in the park. Here we are at the park, and my friend began telling me how accomplished I am and how the hand of God is on my life. As she continued to talk, I broke down and said, "I understand but I'm tired". She held me at that moment and said, "I know and it's ok" as my tears continued to fall.

What I've learned that I hope blesses you is, yes, you can be strong, but it is ok to simply be tired. Have your moment to release, meaning to cry out and scream if you have to, and release with someone of wisdom, who has your greatest interest in mind. It is ok to cry, scream, and simply be human. You are still stronger as your release.

Let God be God and know that in all of your greatness, it's ok to simply be tired. Every strong person deserves to press the pause button and reset.

Find your pause button today and use it as needed. God made you beautiful and with an abundance of life. Cherish your mind, body, and spirit. Your past will be proud of you. Your present will honor you and your future will thank you. Take care of YOU and know that it is ok to be tired; just pause.

Day 12: Our words have power: I CAN DO THIS!

Death and life are in the power of the tongue: and they that love it shall eat the fruit thereof.
~Proverbs 18:21 KJV

Today, speak words of life and strength over YOURSELF: "I am loved. I am strong. I am a winner. I have faith bigger than my diagnosis. I am cherished. God loves me. I CAN DO THIS! I have a purpose. I can do this! I am royalty. I am beautiful. I am a priority. I am resilient. I CAN DO THIS! I am not defeated. I am strong and I will overcome my challenges. I am wise. God gave me this life to live in abundance. I will use my voice to impact lives. I am a trailblazer. I am a world changer. Life, love, and freedom are my reality. I CAN DO THIS! I am not defeated. My diagnosis does not define me. I am beautiful. I am powerful. MY life is in the hands of God. My trust is in God. All things work together for the good of them that love the Lord. I am called to change lives. My testimony is my assignment. My life is of purpose. My name is victorious. I CAN DO THIS!"

Day 13: Yield

But they that wait upon the LORD shall renew their strength; they shall mount up with wings as eagles; they shall run, and not be weary; and they shall walk, and not faint.

~Isaiah 40:31 KJV

Pray With Purpose

Walk With Purpose

Speak With Purpose

Live With Purpose

Eat With Purpose

Work With Purpose

Anything that you do daily, serves a purpose. Let's Make it Great!

Day 14: Thank You Lord for Time

And let us not be weary in well doing: for in due season we shall reap, if we faint not. ~Galatians 6:9 KJV

There's a timing for everything under the sun. But what is the purpose of these moments? Use today as a time to reflect on the now, by placing things in position for the days ahead. What does that mean? God gives us time throughout the day to first and most importantly seek Him before we do anything. Seeking God isn't simply to gather instructions, but to also talk to Him, cry out and talk things through. A moment in time that we have each day, will never be repeated the same way. Every second is uniquely tailored for that moment. I am thankful that God is blessing you with specific moments in your day that are touched by His purpose of time. In all the busyness that your day may include, stop to reflect on time, inhale, exhale and cherish each moment. Be productive, but understand that the timing of God is well.

Day 15: Take a Break

Be careful for nothing; but in everything by prayer and supplication with thanksgiving let your requests be made known unto God. And the peace of God, which passeth all understanding, shall keep your hearts and minds through Christ Jesus. Finally, brethren, whatsoever things are true, whatsoever things are honest, whatsoever things are just, whatsoever things are pure, whatsoever things are lovely, whatsoever things are of good report; if there be any virtue, and if there be any praise, think on these things. ~Philippians 4:6-8 KJV

Breathe. Pause. Rest. Regroup.

Find your quiet space and take a break as many times as you may need to. You are a priority.

Day 16: My Presence

You will show me the way of life, granting me the joy of your presence and the pleasures of living with you forever. ~Psalm 16:11 NLT

Where the Spirit of the Lord is, there is liberty. Today is a day of discovery and embracing the continued peace of God, in every conversation and decision that you encounter. The joy of the Lord is your strength, and you are a walking creation directly from His hand. You are of joy and peace, and wherever you go throughout your day, it will meet you. Enjoy each moment of your day by thanking God for His peace that surpasses all understanding and walk in the truth that God is present. In the pain, the presence of God is with you. During the appointments, the peace of God is with you. In His presence, you are victorious.

Day 17: Your Posture of Praise in your Day

I will bless the Lord at all times; his praise shall continually be in my mouth.

~ Psalm 34:1 KJV

Is it easy to have positive thoughts all the time during this journey? If you allow me to be transparent with you, for me, that was not the case 100% of the time. Yes, depressive thoughts will come. Yes, moments of uncertainty about the future rose. What I know to be true is, God knows the moments when you will feel discouraged. God knows each moment when your faith will falter. However, the blessing in it is He is not too far. There is a process of faith-building that occurs during this journey, that you may not have had before the diagnosis and God knew that too. There will come times when despite how it feels, you will bless the Lord. Despite how your flesh may feel, allow praises, peace, and love to flow from you. As I've mentioned before, be gentle with yourself and trust God with your day today. I will bless the Lord at all times and His praise shall continually be in my mouth. There will come a time when the peace of God will rest in your mind, body and spirit; and praises will flow from your mouth. Praise is a weapon against the enemy, who desires for you to be defeated spiritually and mentally during this journey. He will not win, and this is a day to rejoice, grow, and develop. Praise God throughout your day and receive Matthew 11:28-30, "Come unto me, all ye that labour and are heavy laden, and I will give you rest. Take my yoke upon you, and learn of me; for I am meek and lowly in heart: and ye shall find rest unto your souls. For my yoke is easy, and my burden is light." The Joy of the Lord is your strength.

Day 18: Pray with Power and Move with Authority

For the weapons of our warfare are not carnal but mighty through God to the pulling down of strongholds. Casting down imaginations, and every high thing that exalteth itself against the knowledge of God and brining into captivity every thought to the obedience of Christ.

~2 Corinthians 10:4-5 KJV

As you go throughout your day, I pray that you to remember that you are the joint heirs with Christ of the authority of God. Your weapon is the word of God. Prayer, faith, and application are the activation of the word of God in your life. You have the authority through Christ to cast down every toxic thought that may try to overpower you today. You have the authority through Christ to bring every thought into captivity to the obedience of Christ. Let the Lord be the shoulder that you lean on today and walk in authority, remembering that you are the joint heirs of God with Christ!

Day 19: Thoughts

Finally, brethren, whatsoever things are true, whatsoever things are honest, whatsoever things are just, whatsoever things are pure, whatsoever things are lovely, whatsoever things are of good report; if there be any virtue, and if there be any praise, think on these things. ~Philippians 4:8 KJV

Despite what you are facing, if you desire to be happy and express your happy moments, do so freely. I would like to remind you that if you chose to be hopeful, you have every right to do so and as I've mentioned, you are the top priority. Sadly, some think negatively about breast cancer and today, I admonish you to pay attention to who those people are and provide whatever distance that you deem necessary. If you love people, keep showing love. If you are an encourager, keep encouraging people. If you just love helping others, continue changing lives. Establish boundaries and know where to place them. Never allow someone's negative views to prevent you from spreading peace to others. Never allow the negativity of someone to cause you to doubt yourself. Do what you love and do it unapologetically and intentionally. Do what is in your heart with great purpose.

After receiving my diagnosis, I did not share the news with many people. However, when I was ready to share it publicly, I did. I was told not to share my diagnosis because people would pray negative things about me. However, when you understand your purpose and who leads your path, you don't have to live in fear. In my sharing, I was able to encourage other women. In this journey, you will discover so much confidence and divine purpose within you.

Day 20: Moving Forward

The Lord directs the steps of the godly. He delights in every detail of their lives. ~Psalm 37:23 NLT

The thoughts of moving forward are some of the most challenging things for some during this journey. Moving forward. When I think about Moving Forward, I think about how you and I take steps by walking. Deciding to lift one foot after the other, first begins in the mind. You've focused on a target or destination, and you've made the decision to take one foot and step one after the other, and you will not stop until you have reached your endpoint. What happens when you're walking in this journey called life to reach your destination and life goals, and an obstacle that requires you to stop and make adjustments to your life? This journey includes many moments of having to stop, adjust, and refocus. What I want to encourage you with today is despite what obstacles that come into your path today, that if you must stop and refocus, do it. Moving forward takes courage and determination. You have it in you to step forward today and in the days ahead. One day and one step at a time.

Day 21: New Season

Trust in the Lord with all thine heart; and lean not unto thine own understanding. In all thy ways acknowledge him, and he shall direct thy paths. ~Proverbs 3:5-6 KJV

When facing an experience in your life that is life-altering, the question at most times is, "Lord, Why Me, Why Me?" In facing my diagnosis, and my challenges with depression throughout my life I asked, *God, why me?* Before I realized that I didn't have to live in a mindset and lifestyle of defeat, I began to say "Ok Lord, what are You trying to develop within me? Help me to understand Your purpose behind this." The process for me was hard and challenging because my flesh was tired. After I decided to fight regardless of what would happen, I chose to Walk BY Faith in a place that I've never been exposed to. The scripture from Proverbs 23:7, "For as a man thinketh in his heart, so is he…"

Our words can bring us victory and our words can also bring us thoughts of defeat. So, the question may be what's next? What's new for you? The newness that awaits you in the day is another revealing of your strength, and when weakness arises, your strength will come around to stand in the gap. Weakness is another opportunity for strength to be revealed and developed. Don't shy away from any moment of development that this journey brings you. You are victorious and came into this world victorious. Love yourself a little more each day and celebrate everything. There aren't any big or small victories in this journey. Each day that you are determined to fight, even physically when your body says otherwise, that's a victory. I celebrate you and I am so proud of you! The journey comes with two major options in terms of the direction of our lives, and we chose the option to live. You never know how strong you are, until being strong is the only option that you have. Even in weakness, you are strong. Be gentle with yourself and remember that you are God's beloved, and your fight and your strength are blessing many people more than you know. I love you so much!

~Taneya

About the Author

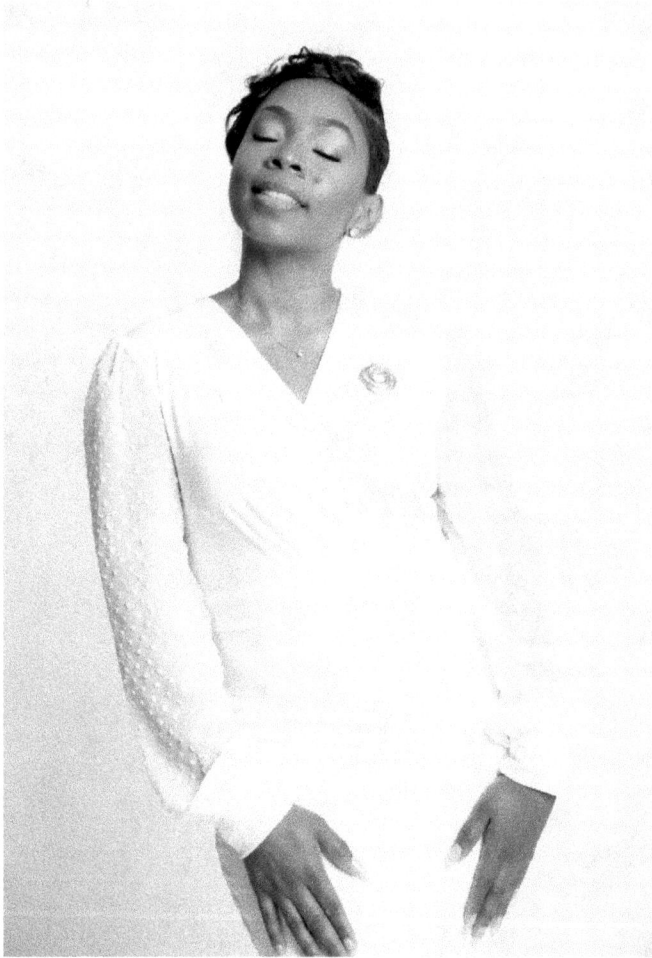

Taneya Pair

Taneya Pair is a native of Washington, DC. Throughout her life's journey, Taneya has remained active in her purpose which began as early as 5 years old. As a child, Taneya discovered her passion for nurturing and assisting others while facing challenging times in their lives. Taneya is a graduate of Trinity Washington University with a Masters in Clinical Mental Health Counseling.

Taneya has the heart of a servant and dedicates her days to serve God and His people within her church, career, and community within various capacities. Taneya is an author, owner of *Cherish* handmade jewelry, Member of *Federal Women's Program, Legislative Ambassador of American Cancer Society CAN* and Founder of *Victorious Over Depression* and *Cherish The Steps Challenge* which focuses on depression awareness. She has had the privilege of speaking on various podcasts, TV and radio shows, and conferences that focused on Breast Cancer Awareness and Mental Health , Women and Youth Empowerment and Dating with Purpose.

Lastly, Ms. Pair enjoys serving within her church at First Baptist Church of Highland Park under the direction of Dr. Henry P. Davis III , along with serving within her communities in various capacities.

www.ingramcontent.com/pod-product-compliance
Lightning Source LLC
Chambersburg PA
CBHW072137270326
41931CB00010B/1789